A Children's Story and Coloring Book

Terry's Journey to
CF LAND

Navigating the Adventures of Cystic Fibrosis

Written by Terry Gene Wright

Illustrated by Dwight Stegall, Jr

Carpenter's Son Publishing

Terry's Journey to CF Land

©2020 by Terry Gene Wright

Published by Clovercroft Publishing, Franklin, Tennessee
www.clovercroftpublishing.com

Edited by Andrew Toy

Cover and Interior Design by Suzanne Lawing

Illustrations by Dwight Stegall, Jr

ISBN: 978-1-950892-77-8

Printed in the United States of America

Acknowledgements

This book is dedicated to cystic fibrosis patients around the world and their families, loved ones, supporters, caretakers, and healthcare providers. And to my wonderful mother, Rose Wright, who has been tirelessly by my side with loving tender care since birth; and my beautiful wife, partner, and Butterbean, Michele Wright, who has lovingly, unselfishly, and faithfully stood with me and supported me for the past twenty-plus years. Everything I am is because of their love! Thank you for being an invaluable part of my continual CF journey!

"No matter what comes your way, don't lose hope, believe in your strength, and always hold on to your faith for a better you and the betterment of others."

~Terry Gene Wright

Special thanks to the following for their financial support: National Organization of African Americans with Cystic Fibrosis (NOAACF); My Water Buddy Foundation; Attain Health Foundation; the Community of Red Lodge, Montana; and Vertex Pharmaceuticals. And heartfelt appreciation to: Kelly Bullington, Arkansas-West Tennessee Chapter of the Cystic Fibrosis Foundation (CFF AR-West TN); John Nash, LCSW; Kat Quinn Porco, MS, CDCES, Attain Health Foundation; Everett Rice; Dwight Stegall, Jr; Siri Vaeth, MSW, Cystic Fibrosis Research, Inc. (CFRI); and Michele R. Wright, Ph.D., My Water Buddy Foundation; alongside everyone from my design and publishing team for your selfless contributions to the journey of this book and graciously helping to successfully bring this project to its long-awaited destination!

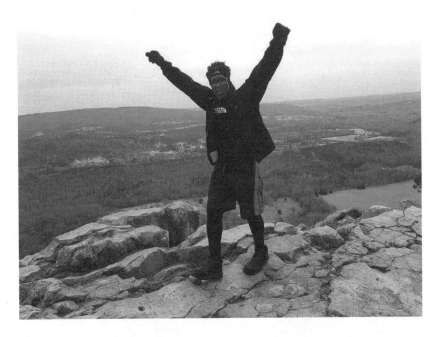

As an African American man living with cystic fibrosis (CF) for 50 years, Terry's story and experiences are very familiar, except that my doctors discovered my CF at the age of 9. Most people with cystic fibrosis endure many challenges, physically and emotionally. They struggle, like most, to find their place, their purpose, and their identity in a confusing world. Living with a rare disease makes the journey even more cumbersome and often allusive, particularly for minorities that may have historically been overlooked. *Terry's Journey to CF Land* is an excellent biographical tale that is lighthearted, but encouraging to other children who live with cystic fibrosis, as well as their families, friends, and loved ones. His optimistic attitude and determination to live the best life he can is a message that every child or adult should hear.

–EVERETT RICE, 50-year-old African American living with cystic fibrosis

Introduction by Michele Wright, Ph.D.

Terry Wright is not only my beloved husband, but my inspiration throughout our 20 years of marriage. At the age of 58, he is a true champion and beacon of hope for individuals suffering from cystic fibrosis.

Following his cystic fibrosis diagnosis at the extraordinary age of 54, Terry has made it his mission to bring a breath of fresh air, hope, and encouragement to his fellow cystic fibrosis sufferers and their loved ones.

I hope that this book uplifts, which is Terry's ultimate hope as well. And I am privileged to be by his side throughout this surreal journey. Enjoy this unique and heartfelt story and coloring book as you join his (our) journey, while conquering and succeeding in yours. The BEST is yet to come!!!

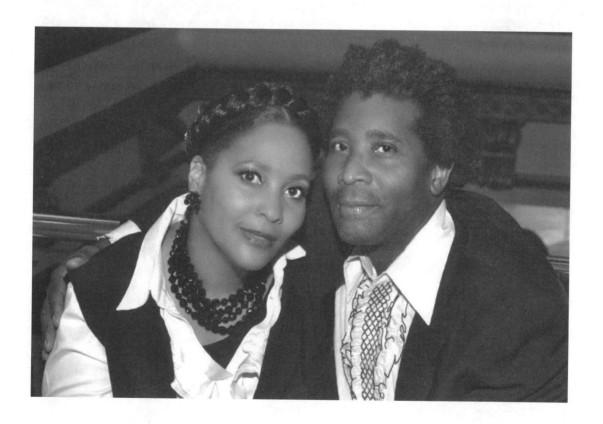

In my role as a medical social worker over the past 18 years, I have had the honor of serving many individuals and their families living with cystic fibrosis (CF). On this journey, there were times when it was clear to me that CF affected people of color, in addition to the people of white European descent. Unfortunately, educational efforts and materials related to living with CF have rarely focused on the experience and needs of black, indigenous, and people of color living with CF. Thanks to the efforts of the National Organization of African Americans with Cystic Fibrosis (NOAACF), this is now changing. Their work will decrease the isolation often experienced by minority groups living with CF as they work to create educational materials and resources that are representative of all people living with CF! Thanks for working to fill a great need!

–**JOHN NASH**, LCSW

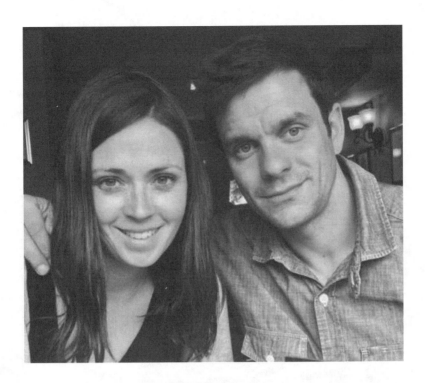

Foreword by Kat Quinn Porco, MS, CDCES

Twelve years ago I walked into the cystic fibrosis community, my child bravely carrying the title. The only word that summed up the complexity of emotions that I embodied was *alone*.

I found myself wading through the overwhelming feelings the only way I knew how: by finding hope. I flooded myself with resources, creating community around illness. I found hope through stories, blogs, and new friendships. And I learned quickly that resources for CF abound . . . if you are white.

All the books, pamphlets, and advertisements in CF are geared toward our race, reminding us that we are supported. However, the minority groups living with CF are left behind to live in our world with little access to supportive resources.

This book is an expression of the tenacity and supreme hope that fills both Terry and Michele. I could not be more honored to know them and see this project come to fruition.

I anxiously await the impact this book holds for children living in the racial minority of cystic fibrosis.

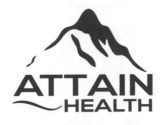

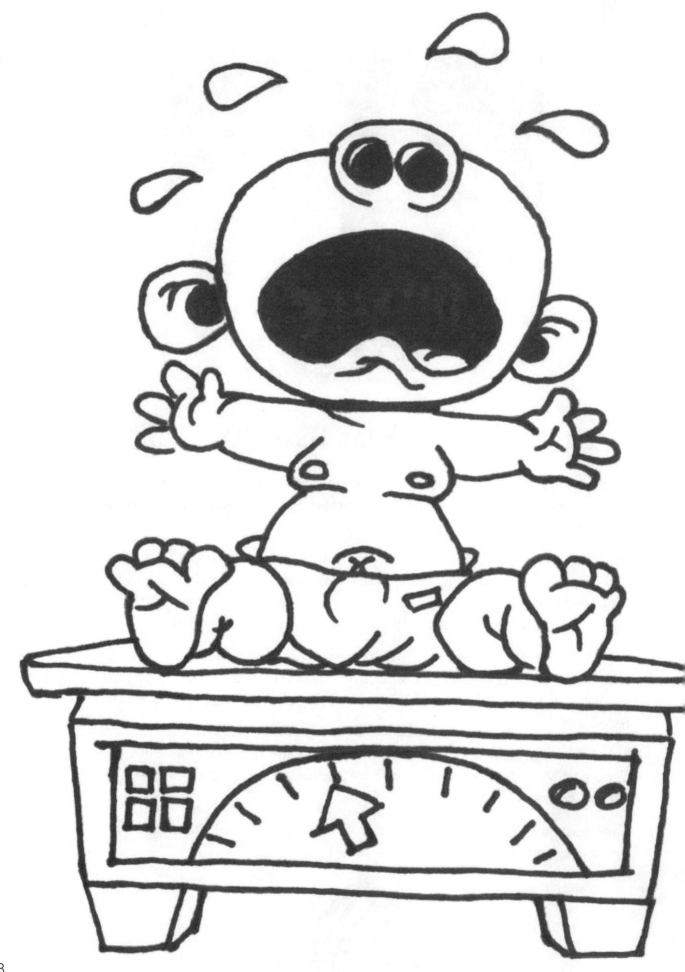

Chapter 1: Breath of Life (Age 0-1)

The doctor looks down and smiles at Mama Rose and hands her a healthy looking baby boy, named Terry. He says, "Congratulations, you just had a sweet bundle of love with a pair of good screaming, healthy lungs." Rose cries and says, "He is perfect, and I am so happy he is well and alert." Terry then stops crying and smiles as he is passed to his daddy, James, who is very proud to hold and snuggle his new baby boy. "He looks just like me," claims James, and then proudly introduces Terry to the rest of his brothers and sisters so that they can admire their youngest sibling as well. Terry feels the love, as his parents prepare to take him home for his new and exciting adventures in life.

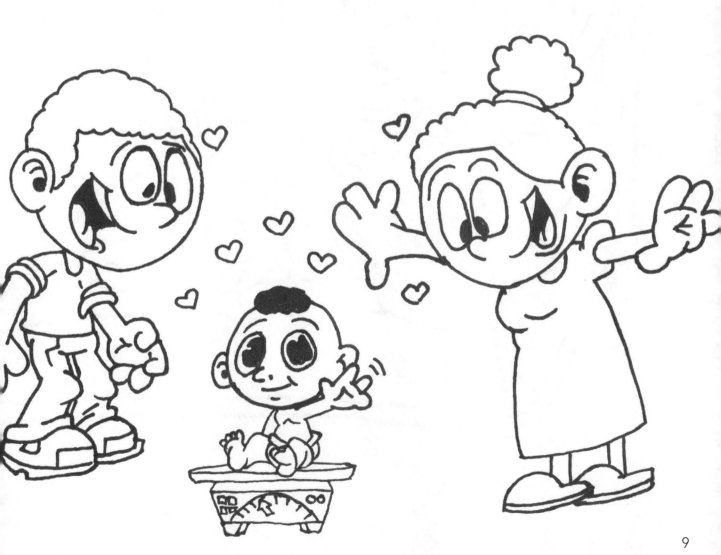

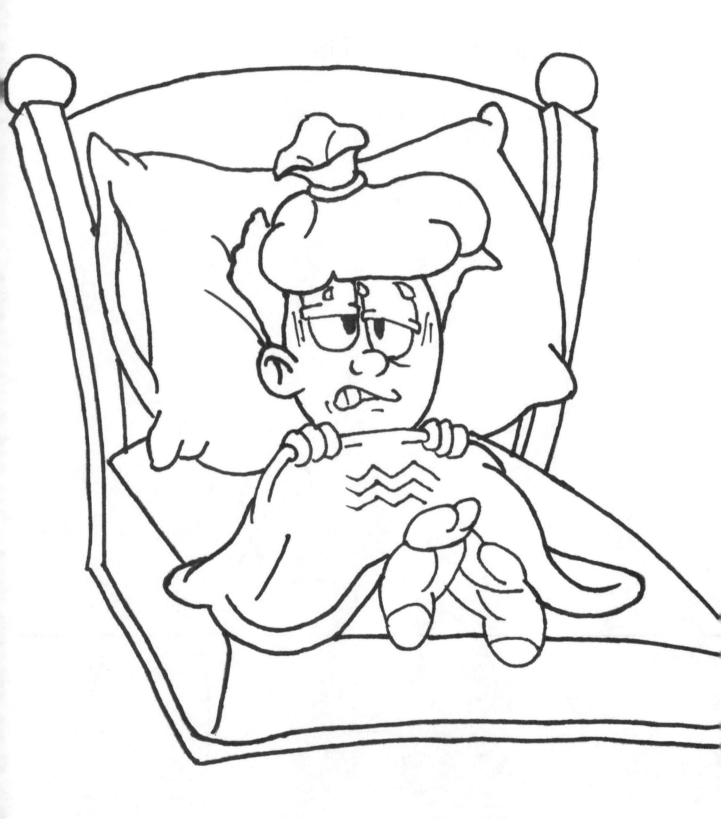

Chapter 2: A Gut Feeling (Age 1-3)

Mama Rose awakes to Terry moaning at two o'clock in the morning. She reaches down in his bed and quickly picks him up. She asks him, "What is wrong, baby?" Terry continues to whimper as he mumbles, "I can't sleep and my tummy hurts, Mama." Mama Rose kisses his forehead and puts him in the bed with her to try to comfort him. The next morning at breakfast, he can't eat and his pain worsens. She then loads him in their 1960s family station wagon and heads to the nearest children's hospital. The doctor admits Terry to the hospital, but assures Rose that Terry has a stomach virus that will pass with time. This will continue to be his untold story throughout his childhood along with countless of hospitalizations and sleepless nights that will follow him throughout his life.

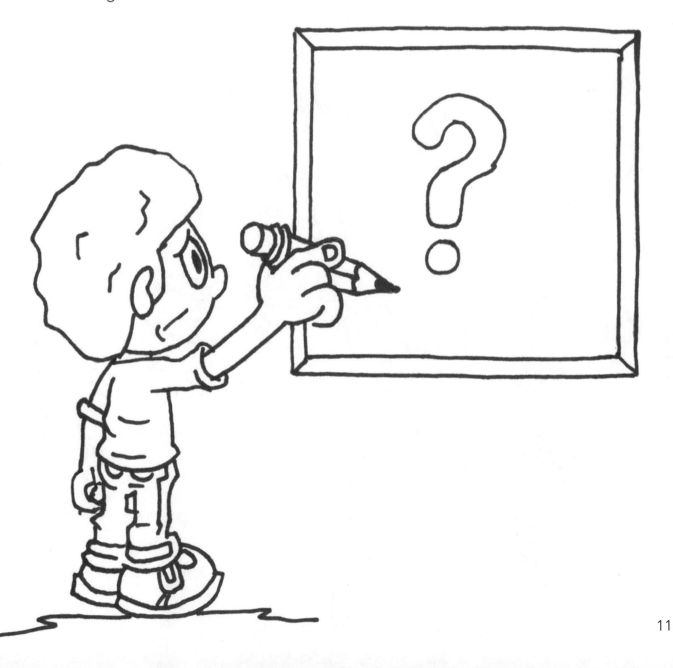

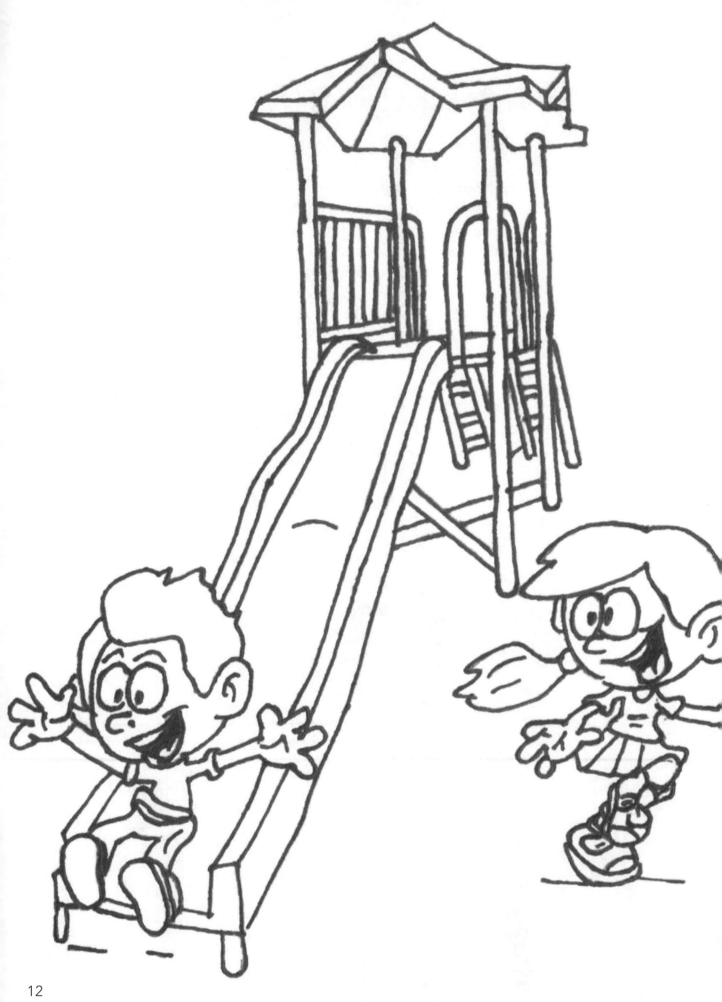

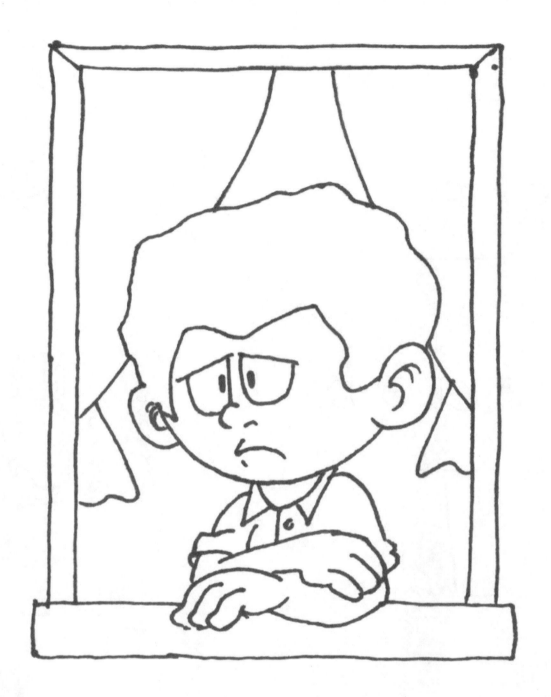

Chapter 3: "Mama, I Want to Play" (Age 3-9)

Mama Rose becomes very protective of her baby boy, who is outgoing in spite of his stomach pains. But Terry sadly looks out the window and is determined to go outside to play with his friends. After begging his mom to let him, she eventually and cautiously lets him go. Terry has so much fun playing with his red wagon, his favorite game of hide & seek, and running around the yard. Rose is also happy when she sees him having so much fun in the sun. She then notices Terry constantly trying to catch his breath. This concerns her enough to take him back to the hospital, where he is diagnosed with childhood asthma, which causes him to miss many days of school. But neither tummy aches nor asthma could keep Terry from playing or stepping up his game. He is determined to be his best in school, sports, and life!

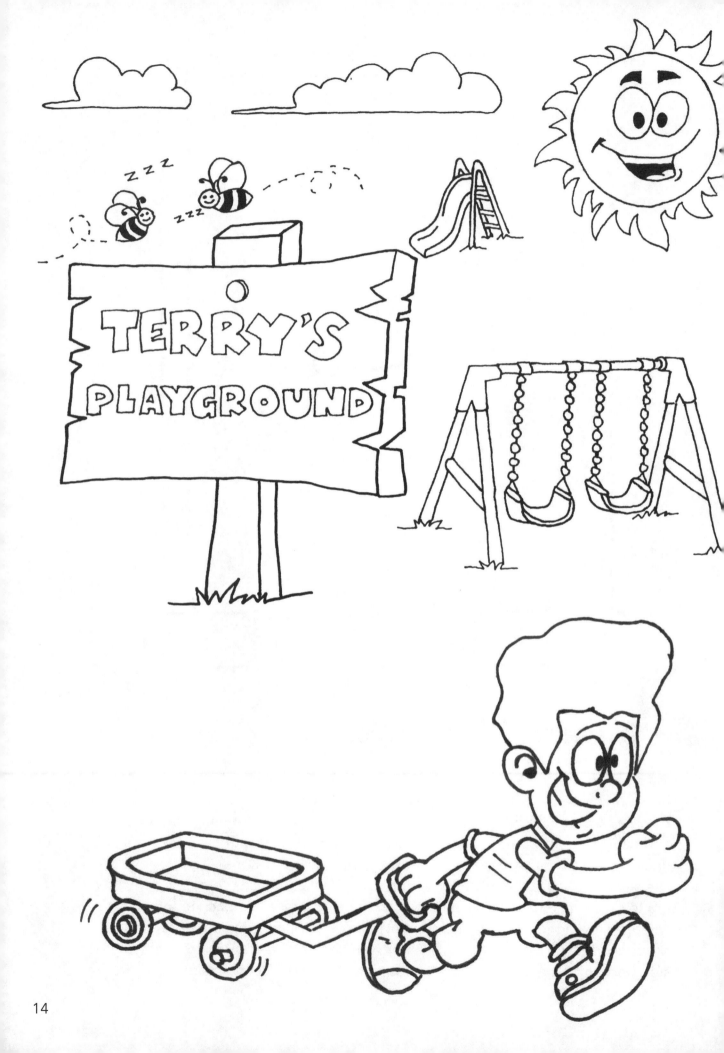

Chapter 4: Winning the Race (Age 9-18)

Terry has lots of energy and develops a love for outdoor sports and physical activity. His favorite game is baseball, because his brother Tony is his teammate, and their dad James is the coach. Unlike his Mama Rose, his dad encourages Terry to play sports as hard as he can and to become more active. Terry is a team favorite and proudly leads his team to multiple victories. He knows how to catch the ball and hit the ball out of the park. He also develops a love for track and field in high school and quickly becomes the fastest of the pack. But Terry keeps a secret from his parents. He continues to have trouble breathing and endures stomach aches. Although he is embarrassed to let his parents or friends know, his sheer determination motivates him to not only finish the race, but win the prize.

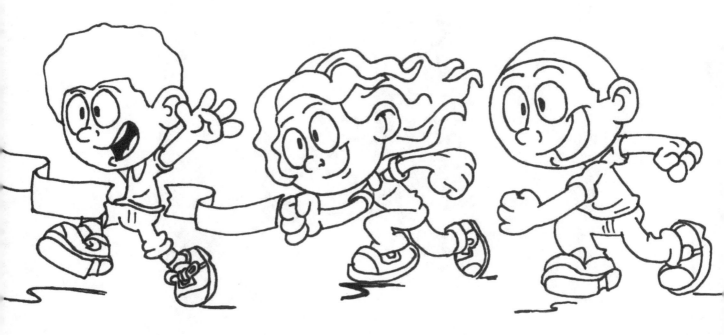

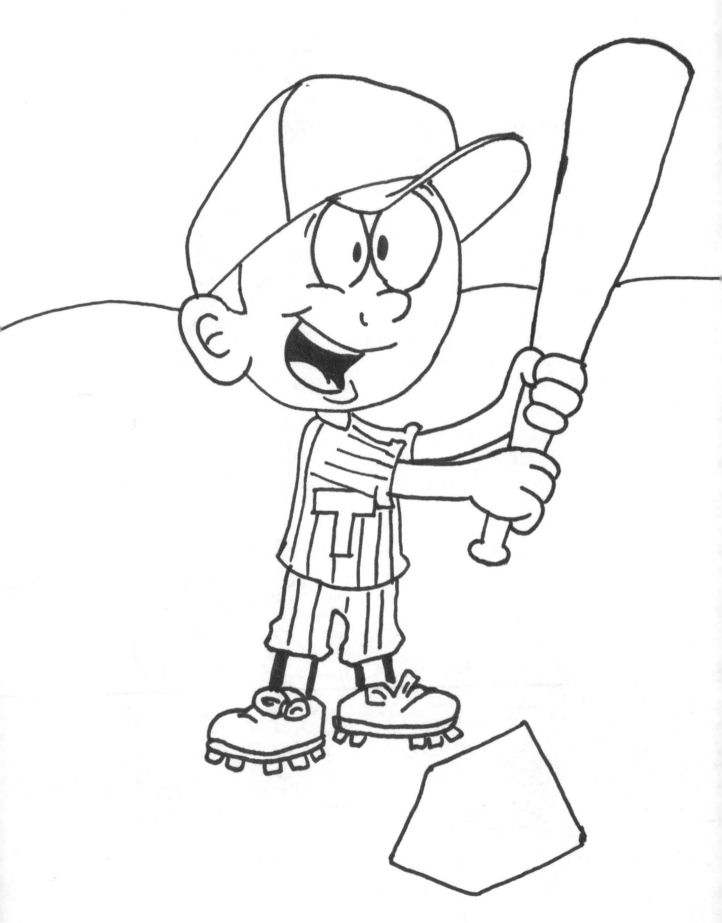

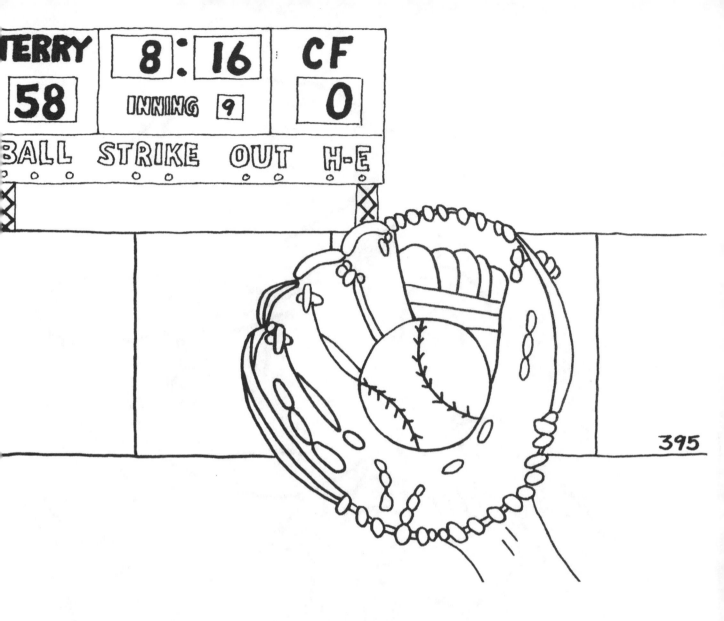

Chapter 5: A Stomach Full (Age 18-26)

Terry continues to excel in sports in spite of his health-related secrets. But the race isn't easy and his journey is becoming more and more difficult to find answers. He is not only experiencing trouble breathing, but he is also revisited by his lifelong stomach aches. Terry cannot understand how he is so different from his other siblings. He tries to work as hard, train as hard, and even run as hard. But his body still suffers. It is a lot for a young man to stomach, which Terry struggles to do. It becomes more and more difficult for him to eat and keep down food. Sometimes, he just lies in bed for days. Oftentimes, he stays at the hospital for weeks. The doctors assure Terry that he has a severe stomach virus, and the cause is undetermined. After a series of hospital visits, admissions, and even a gallbladder removal surgery, Terry knows that he is seriously sick, and he is determined to find answers for better health and a better life.

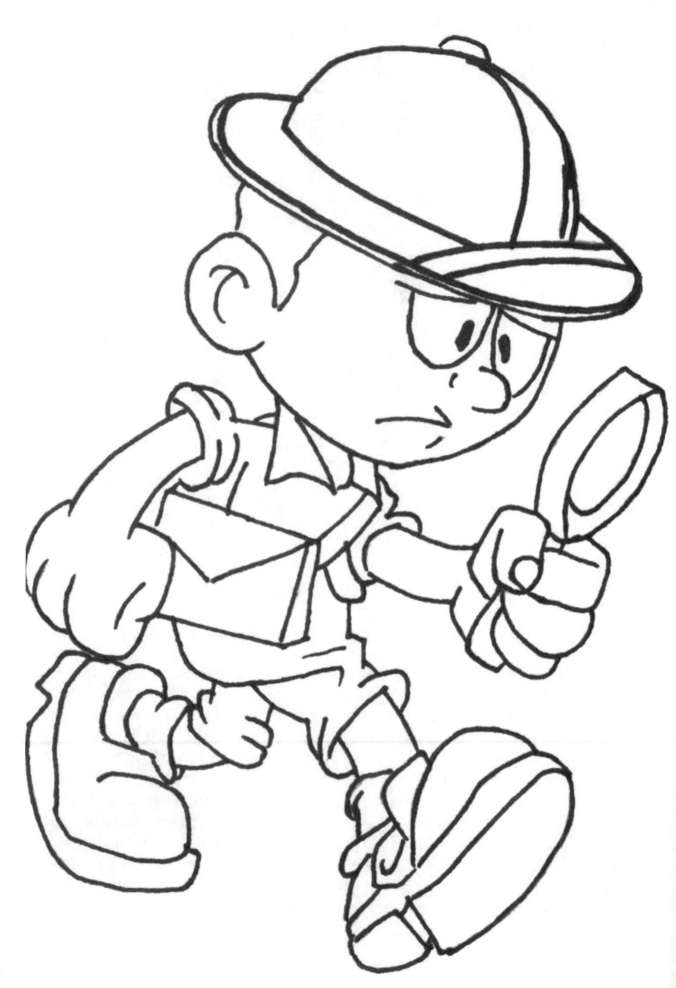

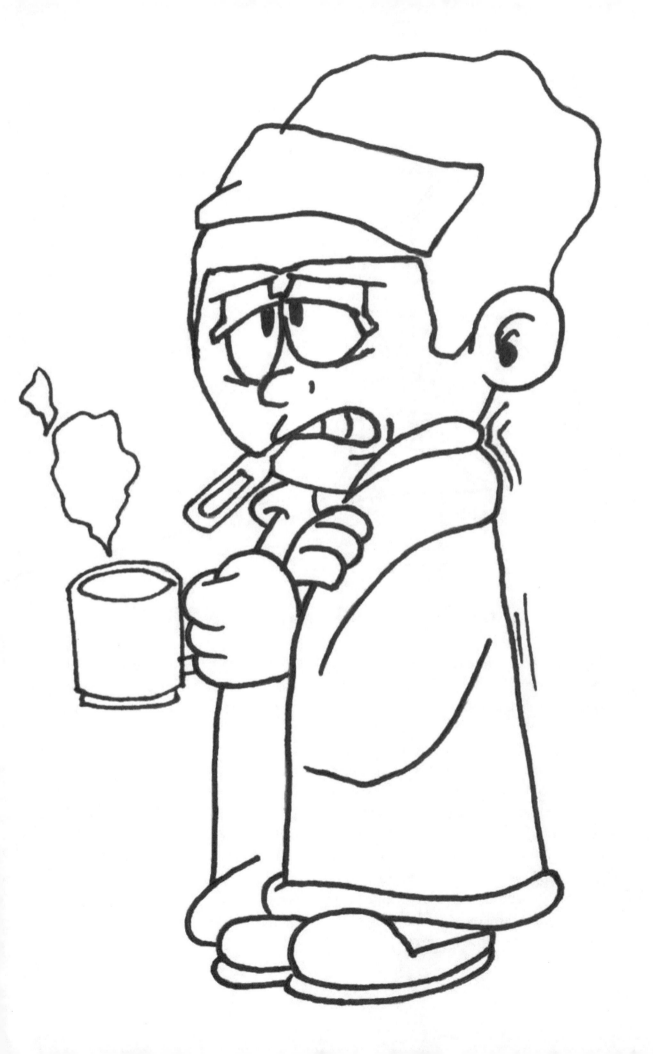

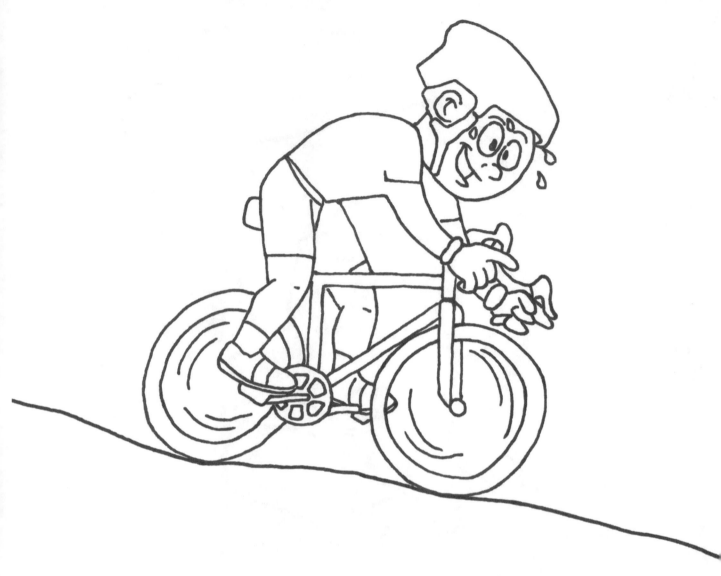

Chapter 6: Inhale/Exhale (Age 26-36)

Terry continues to experience a variety of health challenges, including short-ness of breath, lung infections, persistent coughing, wheezing, migraines, thick glue-like mucus, nasal polyps, fever, unexplained weight loss, nausea, vomiting, visual problems, loss of appetite, salty sweat, and severe stomach problems. Not to mention recurrent pain, fatigue, and depression. After years of many doctor appointments and hospitalizations, Terry is finally diagnosed with chronic pancreatitis, bronchitis, sinusitis, and pneumonia. However, no matter what the nurses, doctors, and hospitals do to help Terry feel better, he only continues to feel worse. But one day, Terry decides that instead of com-plaining, he's going to get up and increase his physical activity and adopt a more positive attitude in life. He starts running again, teaching aerobics, and climbing mountains. He even begins intermediate biking and competing in 100-mile road bike races. Terry is determined to overcome the great pain and to focus on the larger gain.

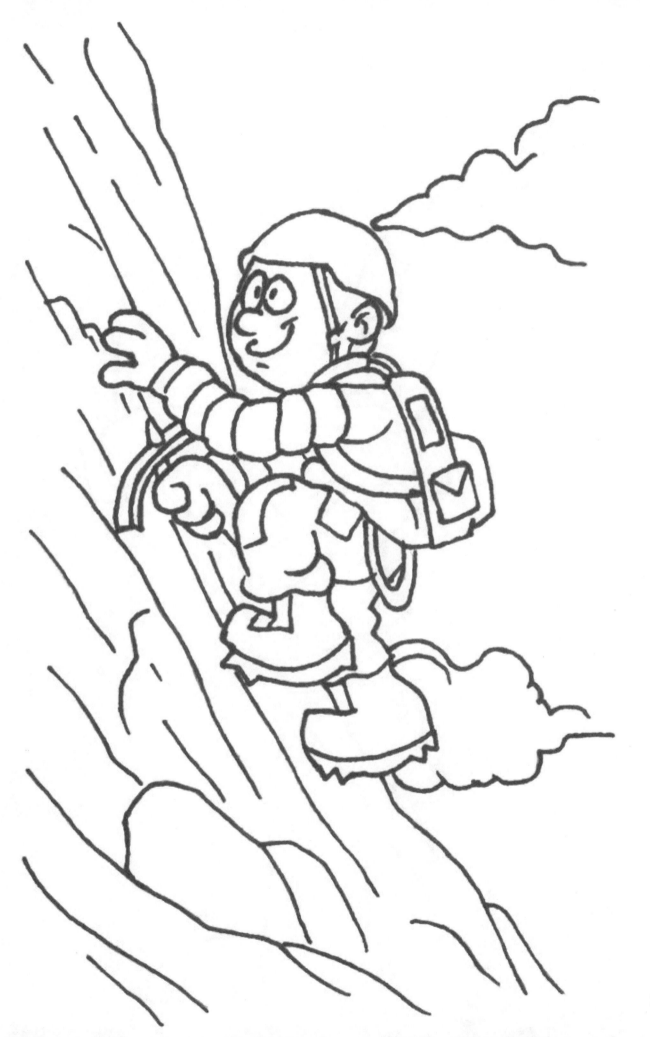

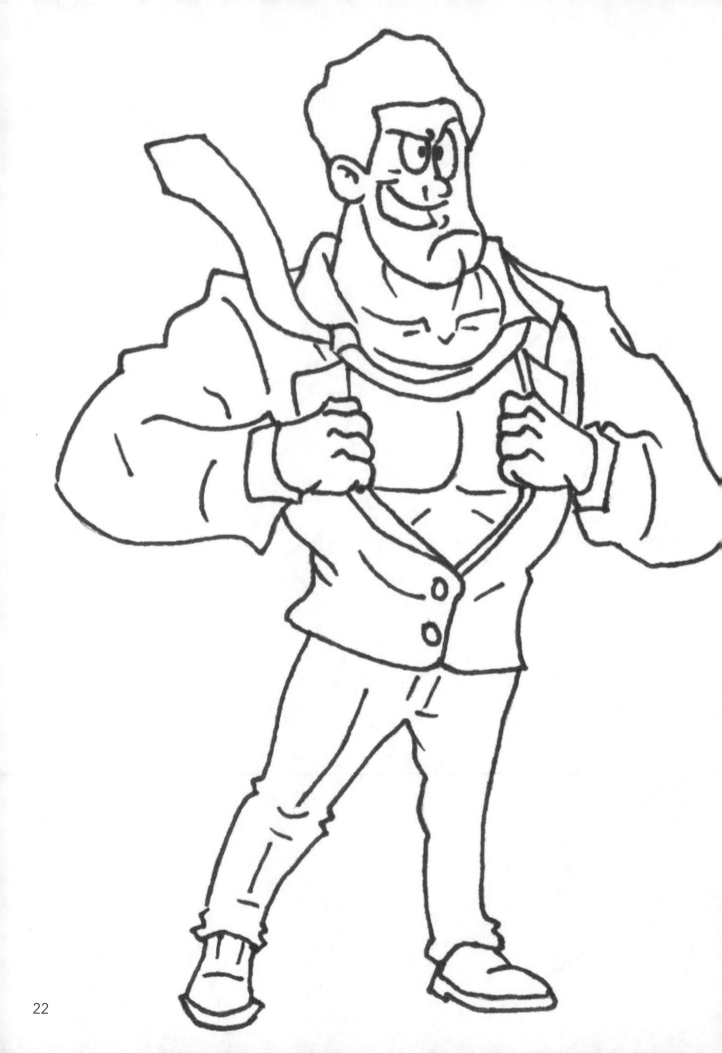

Chapter 7: The Heart of a Super Hero (Age 36-54)

Terry develops the strength of a competitive athlete with the heart of a super hero. He is determined to have a more improved quality of life and health. But little does he know that his change for the better is (W)right around the corner. For his best days are yet to come!

At the age of 37, Terry is introduced to his wife-to-be Michele, a wonderful lady who has actually been called "Wise" since birth. Terry nicknames Michele his "Butterbean" and after a meaningful courtship, they get married. Michele is very concerned about Terry having to go to the emergency room week after week. It is difficult seeing him suffer and being constantly hospitalized. She even watches as he endures a number of sinus and pancreas surgeries. But Terry's Butterbean is fully committed to finding answers and sets out on a mission for him to find better health. After seeing an array of doctors, specialists, and clinics, Terry finally goes to see the doctor who suspects that he has the classic symptoms of cystic fibrosis (CF), which is described by the Cystic Fibrosis Foundation as "a progressive, genetic disease that causes persistent lung infections and limits the ability to breathe over time." Terry is referred back to the same children's hospital, where he spent a lot of his childhood, to be given a sweat test, which measures the amount of chloride (salt) in the sweat. After repeating the results twice, at the atypical age of 54, Terry is finally diagnosed with cystic fibrosis.

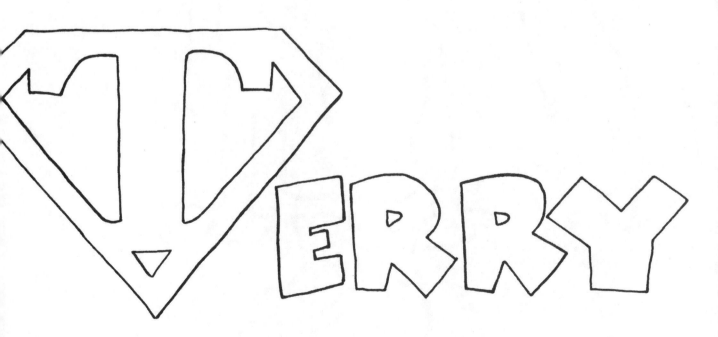

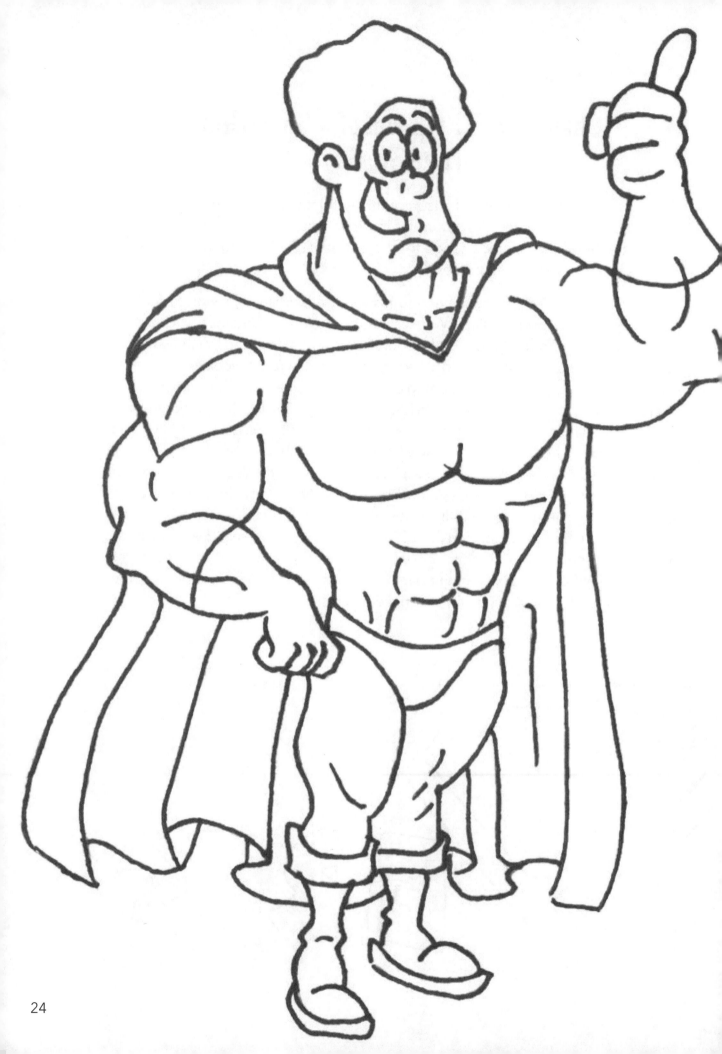

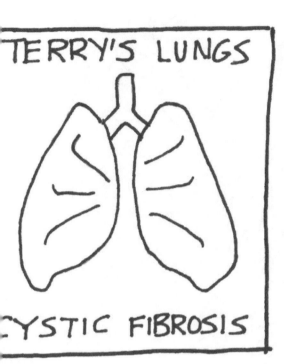

TERRY'S LUNGS

CYSTIC FIBROSIS

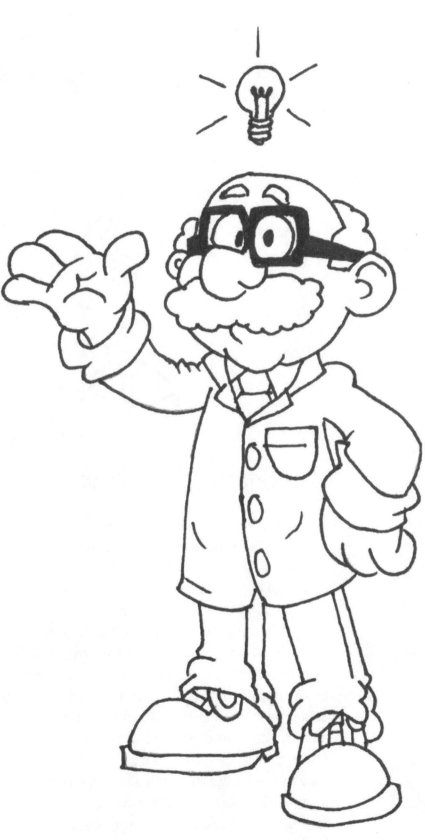

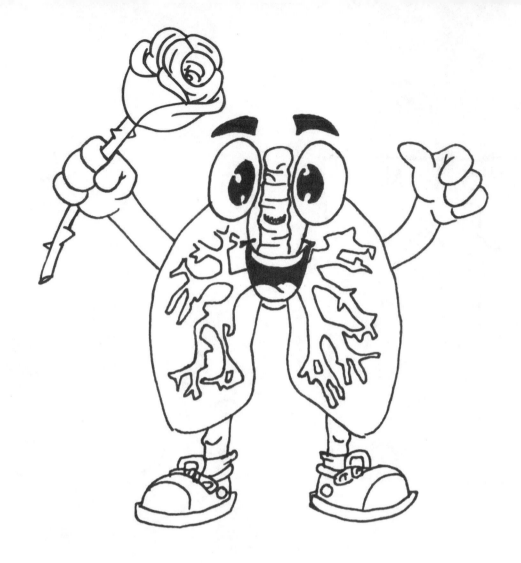

Chapter 8: A New Blue Vest (Age 54-58)

Terry and Michele are happy and relieved to finally have a diagnosis because it actually gives them answers and allows Terry to now receive the correct treatment regimens. This includes a series of breathing treatments, alongside an occasional round of antibiotics, steroids, and antifungals. He also faithfully keeps his health-care medical appointments, fills and takes his prescribed medications, irrigates his sinuses, uses his bronchodilators and inhalers, does his nebulizer treatments, and wears his portable blue CF vest to help facilitate airway clearance and to loosen and thin out the thick mucus genetically caused by cystic fibrosis – all as instructed by his CF care team. Terry believes in the benefits of adherence and knows first-hand how important it is for him to do his daily regimen of care, as instructed, and on time. He also knows the power of a positive attitude and sharing positive vibes. Terry is excited about the difference that his bright and rosy outlook towards cystic fibrosis has made and looks forward to embracing his journey, encouraging others who suffer from cystic fibrosis, and breathing hope for not only today, but for future generations to come. It is his heart's desire. It is his life's mission!

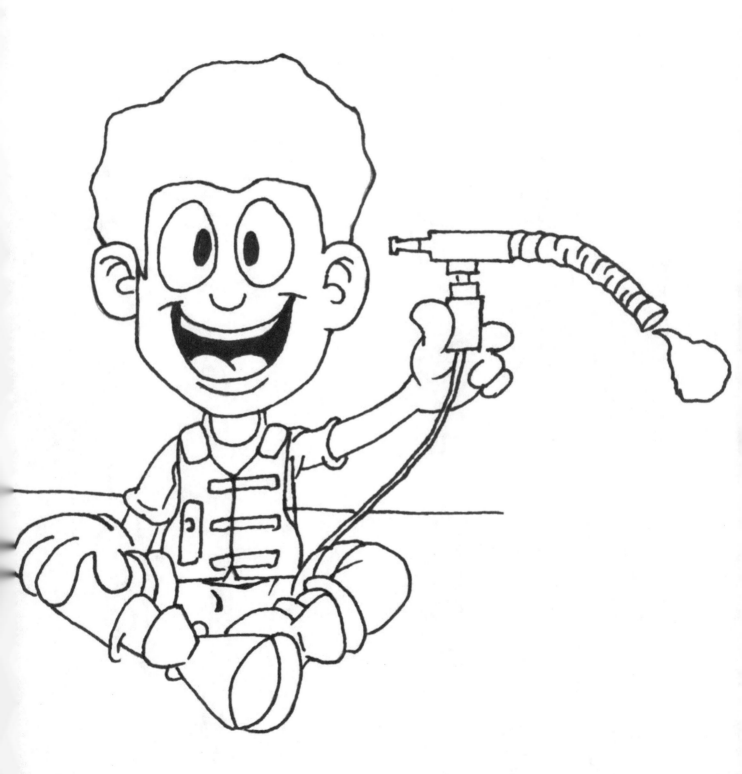

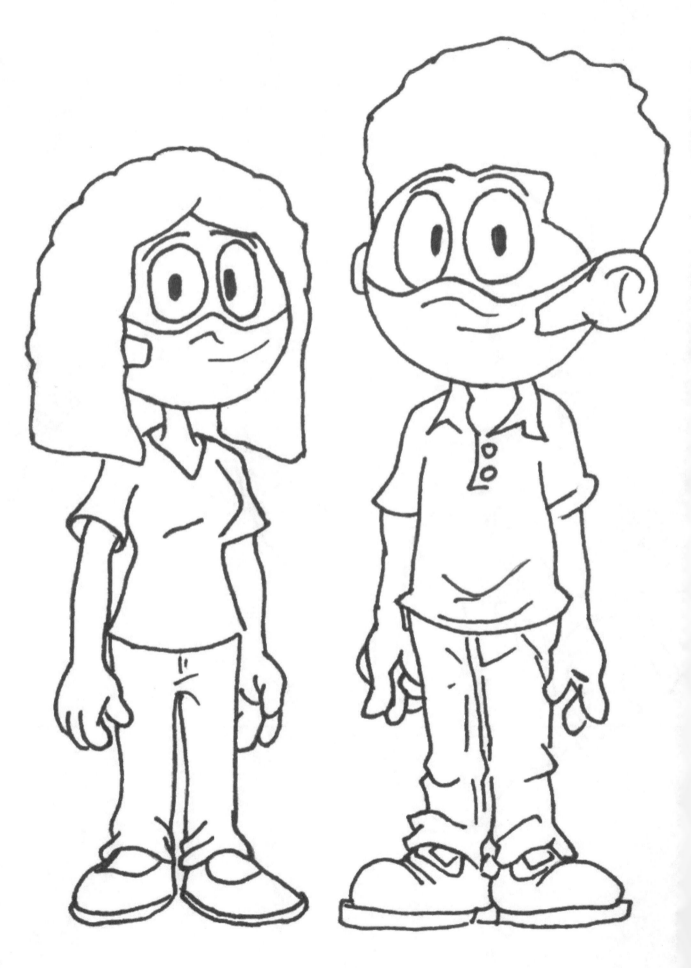

Chapter 9: Breathing Hope
(Age 58 and Older)

Terry has learned to positively seize life one breath at a time, while energetically breathing hope in the lives of others suffering from cystic fibrosis. He understands that he cannot change his CF diagnosis but he can change his outlook for a more positive outcome. Terry likes embracing being a late-age diagnosed CF patient and helping to inspire others who may be afraid, sad, or disappointed with their CF diagnosis. He anticipates and looks forward to a long and prosperous life and one day celebrating his 100th birthday with his Butterbean by his side. He also continues to breath hope in that one day there will be more novel, advanced, and life-changing treatment options for CF'ers and ultimately a CF cure. But until then, Terry will gladly and enthusiastically continue taking his daily medicines; doing his regular treatment regimens; keeping his routine scheduled doctor appointments; and breathing hope, love, and inspiration in the lives of others! It is his duty. It is his purpose. It is, after all, his journey!

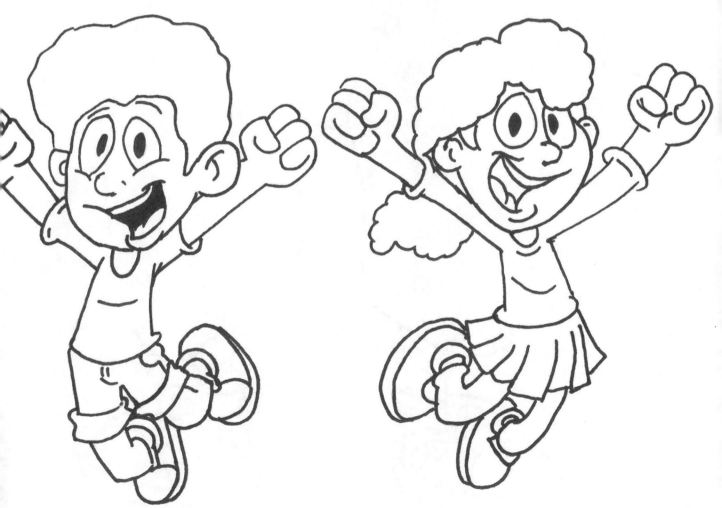

How Are You Feeling Today?

Hi there _____ , (child's name),

Terry really cares about your CF journey and wants to know how you are feeling today! He hopes you are well, happy, and ready to draw and color. Terry's new friend below needs your help, because their face is missing.

So, please help them to be happy by drawing them a face and coloring the rest of their body. And don't forget to share and show your new drawing(s) at www.facebook.com/CFChildrensBook.

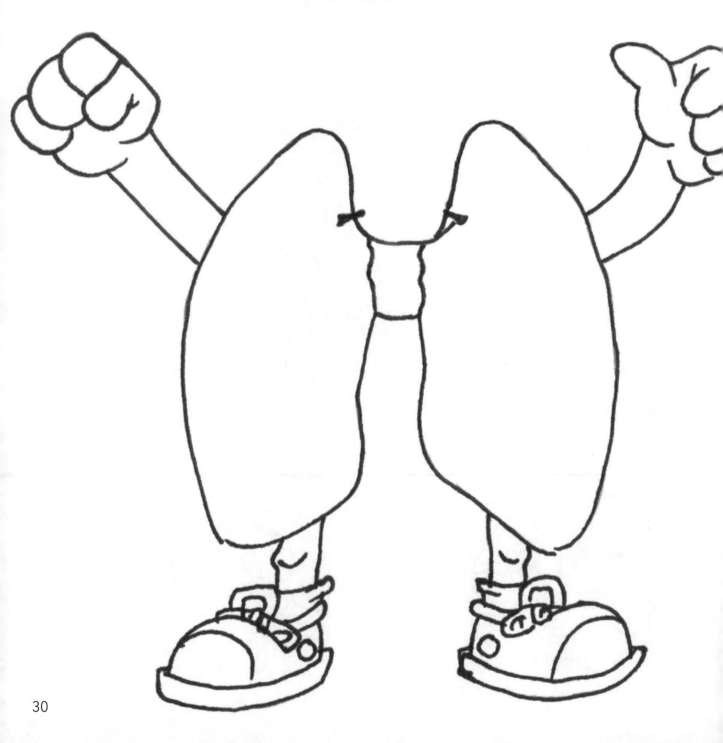

What's Your Favorite Hobby?

Hi there _____ , (child's name),

Can you guess Terry's favorite hobby? (Clue: he loves to eat!)

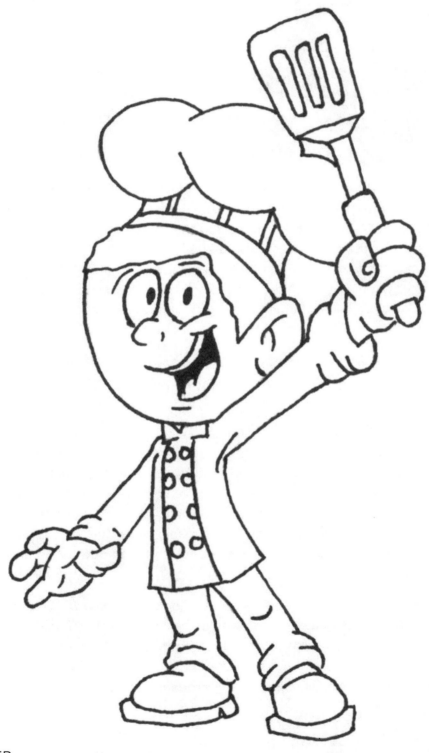

ANSWER:
If you guessed cooking as Terry's favorite hobby, then you are correct! Matter of fact, Terry won the overall Inaugural 2011 Arkansas Cornbread Festival competition.

Terry Wright, Cystic Fibrosis Patient and Advocate

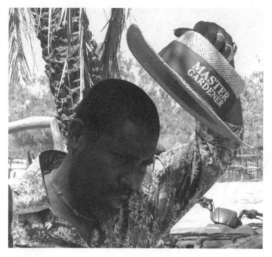

Terry G. Wright is the president and co-founder of the National Organization of African Americans with Cystic Fibrosis (NOAACF), a 501(c)(3) organization with a mission to connect, help build diverse communities, and raise CF Awareness in the African American community and beyond through its national platform. He is the recipient of a 2020 Impact Grant from the Cystic Fibrosis (CF) Foundation (the first person from Arkansas to receive this honor) as well as the 2020 Jacoby Angel Award, the highest award of the CF Roundtable, which is produced by the US Adult Cystic Fibrosis Association (USACFA).

Terry likes to plant seeds of life, love, and hope to help bring change for the better for cystic fibrosis patients, their families, and caretakers. He is an Arkansas dual certified Master Gardener and Master Naturalist. He was elected the 2016 Pulaski County Master Gardner of the Year award winner and a finalist for the 2017 Arkansas Master Gardener of the Year. He completed the standard curriculum in Permaculture Design in 2018. He has also been honored to formerly serve on the North Little Rock Green Committee and Commission on Environmental Efficiency. He has an impressive 38-plus year career as a Certified Personal Fitness Trainer (CPFT).

Today, he wholeheartedly utilizes his deep-rooted passion for gardening, nature, agriculture, horticulture, fitness, nutrition, and health to help individuals from all walks of life to achieve the best in health!

At the age of 54, Terry was unexpectedly diagnosed with cystic fibrosis, a progressive, genetic disease that causes persistent lung infections and limits the ability to breathe over time. This defective gene causes him to endure a thick, sticky buildup of mucus in the lungs, pancreas, and other organs. He has also experienced extensive bacterial infections and recurrent fungal infections including sinusitis, bronchitis, pneumonia, aspergillus, and Burkholderia multivorans. Additionally, he has suffered from chronic pancreatitis due to the mucus preventing the release of digestive enzymes that allow the body to break down food and absorb vital nutrients.

As a consequence of his own life-altering health challenges coupled with the numerous challenging health issues he has witnessed firsthand in the lives of others, Terry is fully committed to utilizing his expertise in gardening, agriculture, horticulture, nutrition, and fitness to help others combat medical issues and achieve a better quality of health and life. Terry lives in North Little Rock, Arkansas with his wife and Butterbean, Dr. Michele R. Wright.

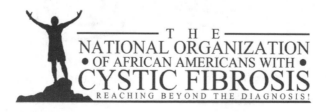